# Praise for *Dear Dr. V...*

"A thoroughly enjoyable book that answers so many questions about life—its trials and tribulations. Marilyn says it like it is!"
> —**Paula Zahn, Emmy Award-winning journalist, television anchor, and host of *On the Case***

"Marilyn Varadi's voice may be silenced, but her words live on. They offer wisdom, warmth, and good old common sense."
> —**Susan Isaacs, *New York Times* best-selling author**

"Right on target... Charming and hits home."
> —**Assemblyman Ed Braunstein, District 26, Bayside, New York**

"Marilyn's voice was always clear, strong, and filled with wisdom."
> —**Linda Carter, PhD, clinical associate professor of psychiatry, NYU Child Study Center**

"Marilyn's confidence, caring, and intellect are evident to her friends and readers alike. She is at her best when being truthful, humorous, and, above all, insightfully sensible."
> —**Leslie and Arnold Gussin**

"Dr. Varadi's warmth and responsiveness to every personal question are so natural and easy. It's a joy to read them!"

"Throughout this time she shined like a beacon through her own dark clouds of adversity and uncertainty while always taking the time to help others with their problems."

"Marilyn's wisdom comes straight from her authentic, learned and loving heart! Her thoughtful insights have helped many over the years."

# Dear Dr. V...

## Dr. Marilyn Varadi

Published by
Varadi Ovarian Initiative
for Cancer Education
(VOICE)

For more information contact Charles G. Rudy
charlesgrudy@hotmail.com
www.voiceforlife.org

Book design by:
Arbor Books, Inc.
www.arborbooks.com

Printed in the United States of America

*Dear Dr. V...*
Dr. Marilyn Varadi

1. Title  2. Author  3. Self-Help

Library of Congress Control Number:  2012912866

ISBN 13: 978-0-615-67051-5

# Table of Contents

# Foreword

Dr. Marilyn Varadi began writing a monthly column, "Relationships in the 21st Century," for the *Tower Times* soon after she moved to North Shore Towers in 1998. With the co-op community serving such an important role in her life, she graciously offered to share her expertise as a renowned psychologist with our readers, offering advice and answering their questions.

Her articles concerned a wide variety of family and relationship issues and quickly became a very popular feature. They are collected here in book form for the first time, and are as insightful today as the day they were published, offering a great deal of wisdom and expertise.

During Marilyn's six-year battle with ovarian cancer that included 160 chemotherapy treatments, her writing for the paper eventually became less prolific, but she continued leading by example. She devoted some of her later columns to describing eloquently what she was going through, and she served as a positive role model for those experiencing similar issues. Throughout this time she shined like a beacon through her own dark clouds of adversity and uncertainty while always taking the time to help others with their problems.

Her disease led her significant other, Charles "Chick" Rudy, to create the Varadi Ovarian Initiative for Cancer Education (VOICE) in 2005, with Marilyn serving as co-chairperson. The *Tower Times* was proud to help promote and report on the organization's annual September dinner-dances, which raised hundreds of thousands of dollars with a mission of promoting early detection of ovarian cancer through education, research, and advocacy. Marilyn and Chick also established the Marilyn Varadi Research Fellowship for Ovarian Cancer Research at the NYU Medical Center in 2007.

Marilyn's untimely death in September 2010 left a chasm in our newspaper and our hearts that is left unfilled. She is deeply missed by our readers and, of course, the publishers of our newspapers.

—Michael Kohn, editor and publisher, *Tower Times*

# Preface

Having had the privilege of knowing and loving Marilyn for almost twenty years, I can say with certainty that she brought a very special brightness into the lives of those she knew. She believed life is to enjoy—don't complicate it. To her, problems were challenges that could, most times, be overcome. Yes, some are more difficult than others, but surely anything is possible. These beliefs permeated her everyday thoughts and actions.

Marilyn's smile and easygoing way made everyone around her feel comfortable. She was never confrontational, and she was always there to listen, understand, and assist. She felt that helping others was a way to grow personally and to make the world a better place in which to live.

Sharing Marilyn's writings with you gives me great joy. Her thoughts and professionalism have helped so many people over the years. We can learn from her responses to the letters she received as they touch on everyday life. Throughout her career she was an advisor to children and adults, grandparents and friends, and helped them cope with the challenges they faced.

Marilyn believed that expressing and not repressing feelings is the most positive way of handling any situation. Not only her patients but her friends looked to her for counseling, advice, and real yet uncomplicated answers to what they saw as problems and dilemmas.

The following pages may answer some questions you have now or have had in the past. This book shows all of us that we are not alone—our problems are not exclusive to us, and most situations are not insurmountable.

A special thanks to the estate of Marilyn Varadi; Lisa, her daughter; and Mike Kohn and the North Shore Towers' *Tower Times* for making the publication of this book possible.

Enjoy reading *Dear Dr. V.*

—Chick Rudy

# Introduction

I was thoroughly charmed by Marilyn's writings for the North Shore *Tower Times* newspaper. Her writings sound exactly like the way Marilyn spoke and thought—so natural, so accessible, so down to earth and useable. From the moment Chick asked me to compose this introduction, I felt truly honored, and memories of Marilyn have been flooding my thoughts, both while awake and while sleeping.

Recently I have been supervising a new psychologist with her first real patient, and Staten Island Mental Health came to mind. That was where Marilyn and I met in 1963. We were both psychology interns. From my point of view, I really lucked out having Marilyn as my co-intern. She was a spot-on New Yorker, and I was a naïve transplant from Philadelphia. Meeting Marilyn was like falling into a warm feather bed in what my father had warned me was a cold, hard environment. Once Marilyn came into my life, I could not relate to my father's fearful warning anymore. She was calm, kind, loyal, stimulating—in other words a beyond-a-doubt good friend.

As we began to see patients, Marilyn was supportive. She had some clinical experience at Queens College with a giant in our field, Dr. Rachel Lauer. So Marilyn helped to allay my fears that I was just wasting my patients' time. She reminded me that merely offering a concerned ear to someone who felt no one ever listened or cared about what she was going through was already doing a mitzvah (helping to repair what is broken).

As the year progressed, Marilyn invited me to meet her family in Brooklyn. She happened to live in an apartment building with another soon-to-be-famous psychologist, Dr. David Singer. He became a preeminent researcher. Through my eyes Marilyn was well connected.

We became a team. Marilyn was the sober one, the thoughtful one, the circumspect person, and I was the impulsive, spontaneous, fun-loving other half. I felt so secure having Marilyn in my life in the big, bad city. I was living with three other girls on 71st Street between First and Second. The kind of security Marilyn gave me is more than anyone could ever pay back.

We both agreed to stay on as research assistants for another year at Staten Island Mental Health because they were doing a fascinating study on premature babies and their subsequent physical and mental development, including the possibility of contracting high blood pressure and hyperactivity. We worked in a very small viewing room while we studied mother-infant interactions through a one-way mirror. The other person in the room was a volatile patient named Nancy Turner (not her real name). She was a woman in her fifties or sixties at the time. Marilyn handled her with a smoothness I found incredible. I watched and marveled at Marilyn on a daily basis. I could not fathom how she did it. Nancy loved Marilyn, and you can imagine how she felt about me from the description I offered of our teamwork early on.

Next I told Marilyn about my dream to continue on for a PhD. She wasn't so sure at the time, but with constant encouragement—some would call it nagging—she finally submitted to joining me on this daunting project. After applying to many very hard to get into schools, Marilyn told me about the PhD program in school psychology at New York University. We both applied and were interviewed by Dr. Gilbert Trachtman, who we discovered was the pied piper, father figure, and adoring uncle to all in the program. Marilyn and I both made the waiting list. One day, in keeping with my lack of self-consciousness at that time, I called Dr. Trachtman to find out if I had gotten of the waiting list and onto the roster of incoming doctoral candidates. He gave me the great news—yes, I had made it. Then, without thinking twice, I asked him if Marilyn had made it, as I would have been heartbroken if she had not. His answer was affirmative. When I told Marilyn we both had been accepted, she was as incredulous that I'd had the chutzpah (courage, nerve, boundary-violation ability) to ask if she had gotten in as I was astounded by how the difficult Nancy Turner had loved Marilyn.

During our studies we developed a group of six friends. We did everything together and supported each other through the trials of pledging for the psychology fraternity. Marilyn had known our good friend Dr. Linda Carter from her Queens College days. There were five women and one man, Dr. Richard Kurtzberg. We all had a joke called the "I Like Richard Test." If the men we dated liked him, we knew the men were deep and not superficial.

Following our earning PhDs, Marilyn and I worked together in a psychological institute that we formed with other people. We saw patients, and we drummed up business by getting doctors and school officials to know about our group. When Marilyn and her husband went to Chile to get their daughter Lisa, she left one couple hanging. I took the case, and when Marilyn finally returned with her beautiful baby girl, she was mad at me for it. This was our only argument in all the years we had known each other.

Of course she was right, as had begun to work with these people, and of course I was right, as I did not know when she would return from Chile and I did not want to offend the physician who had referred the couple to us. (This was my business training from Charles Singer, whom I mentioned earlier: always keep the customer happy.) Within days Marilyn and I made up and never misconnected again for all the years we knew each other.

Very soon after Lisa arrived, Marilyn moved to Great Neck. Marilyn then became a school psychologist and spent her career working with the students, staff, and faculty in New York public schools. She found it very gratifying, as she was able to help many traumatized children, supervise staff, and live a calm, predictable life.

Unfortunately John died at a young age, leaving Marilyn a widow. This was where Chick entered the picture. He was the most supportive, reliable, loving friend and life partner Marilyn could ever have hoped to find. They had many years together in health.

Chick kept the boat on a steady, even keel. In a way he played the part in this stage of Marilyn's life that she had offered to me when I'd first moved to New York City. The expression "what goes around comes around" really seems to fit this scenario.

Then Marilyn got sick. And both she and Chick took a miserable experience and turned it into the most admirable creation anyone could have imagined: a research fund for early detection of ovarian cancer. But Marilyn has always been like that, making something good out of a dark experience. She was so lucky to have met a man who shared her character structure. They were the most compatible, loving couple, and an inspiration to all who knew them.

Now, whenever I drive past Marilyn's building on the Long Island Expressway, I feel the pain of her loss. It is so hard to absorb that she is only with us in spirit—though it is a very strong spirit. But that is life, and eventually it will happen to all of us.

So, farewell, my dear friend. What a treasure to have met you when I was so young and to have kept our friendship going all those years.

—Bonnie Jacobson, PhD, author and director,
New York Institute for Psychological Change

# The Way We Live Now: Relationships in the 21st Century

Many of us long for the good old days when life seemed easy and relationships were less complicated. As we live longer, lose spouses, and/or become part of the divorce statistics, at least half of us now have blended families. It must have been a psychologist or family therapist who coined the term *blended family*, since being a stepmother conjures up negative thoughts of Cinderella.

It's much more complicated than the Brady Bunch. For example you may be widowed or divorced and in a new marriage—a second or third. Or you may have a significant other who you may or may not live with. Of course your spouse or significant other has children, making you a stepparent and perhaps a stepgrandparent.

Add to that your children, who may have divorced and remarried, your ex-daughter-in-law, and her new spouse. There probably are grandchildren and stepgrandchildren in this blended family.

To complicate matters, your second spouse may be deceased, but you may maintain relationships with your stepchildren and stepgrandchildren even after you marry again. There are even-more complex family ties that we can note, but you certainly get the picture—or live it.

It was easy planning holiday dinners years ago—do we serve brisket or turkey? Buying holiday gifts, remembering birthdays, and figuring out the protocol at family gatherings now require a new book of etiquette.

In this monthly column I hope to provide some guidance in complex family or personal matters, and it is intended to answer questions written to me or the editor of the *Tower Times*.

—M.V.

# Holidays, Weddings, and Other Blessed Events

*I am dreading Chanukah because I feel I am expected to buy gifts for my new stepgrand-children. They live with my son and his new wife, and I don't know them well. I also don't want to spend as much on them as I spend on my son's own children.*
—Gift-Giving Grandma,
Building 2

Giving should never feel like an obligation but should be a gesture of love and caring. While you don't know these children yet, they are now a part of your extended family; they are your son's stepchildren and your grandchildren's stepbrothers and stepsisters. Thus you will probably spend time with them, and hopefully you will develop positive relationships with them. You can become a beloved elder with non-biologically related people, and in fact these relationships are often less emotionally charged and more fun. There is always enough love for everyone, and with your concern you will be setting a good example of acceptance for your child and grandchildren. Of course be sensitive to possible competitiveness with your grandchildren.

On the practical side, you can confer with your son and new daughter-in-law about the interests of these stepgrandchildren and choose gifts that are age-appropriate, personal, and meaningful rather than just expensive. Perhaps special outing alone to museums or sporting events will also be an opportunities for you to get to know these children apart from the rest of the family. If you have bought your grandchildren one or more expensive holiday gifts, be discrete and give the extra gifts in private, and give the less-costly gifts in front of the stepsiblings.

―――

*My wife makes a wonderful Thanksgiving dinner for her adult children and my adult children and grandchildren. My children bring flowers, desserts, etc., and her children come empty-handed. I know it sounds petty, but I am resentful. What do you think?*
—Looking at the Little Details,
Building 1

Don't lose sight of what is most important: you are lucky to have a large family with whom to celebrate holidays. Many of your neighbors have children living far away or spouses who don't entertain the large, blended and extended family.

Each family has its own customs, such as bringing part of the meal or helping in the kitchen. Your children are thoughtful to bring gifts, and as stepchildren of your wife they may feel especially appreciative of her efforts. Her own children may take her hospitality for granted. If it bothers your wife, it's up to her to say something to her children. If your children are annoyed that other are not bringing gifts, they may choose not to bring something next time. Instead they can help with cleanup, etc. I caution you to tread lightly and not be judgmental in this situation. If you let others know how you feel about what you perceive as an inequity, this may cause rifts in the family. Perhaps you should reflect on what may really be bothering you; perhaps some other resentment in the relationships needs to be addressed.

―――

*As Mother's Day approaches, I find myself wondering if the role of mother to my adult children must be as intense and involved as it was when my two daughters were living*

*at home. To be more specific, my younger daughter has confided in me about an issue she has with her sister. She is asking that I intervene on her behalf. What do you suggest?*
—Ready to Cut the Apron Strings,
Building 2

Do I see sibling rivalry and birth order issues rearing their ugly heads? While being a mother is a lifelong job and there may be inherent responsibilities that come with the territory, in this scenario your role should be very limited.

You are being placed in a no-win situation. How can you take sides, even if you agree with your younger daughter given the facts she presents? As you know there are two sides to the story, and there may be some distortion on your daughter's part, based upon the long history between the two girls. I am sure if you ask your older daughter about the incident she might not even remember it, or she will have a totally different perception of the matter. But don't get involved in any direct way.

On the other hand, you can serve as a sounding board for your younger daughter by hearing her out, asking some nonthreatening questions, and perhaps pointing out something that may be relevant to the matter. Being the younger sister may mean she feels unable to stand up to her big sister, and as young girls they asked Mommy to intervene and settle their disputes.

You must encourage your daughter to talk directly to her sister, preferably in person with no other family around. In this way, hopefully, they can clear the air so they will not hold grudges and they can continue their relationship. You might help her communicate in a way that is not accusatory or judgmental. Conversations that are accusatory and bring up past grievances can only lead to defensiveness and hard feelings. You certainly don' t want a cold war at your Mother' s Day dinner.

Most importantly you are empowering your daughter, who obviously feels insecure in dealing with her sister. She is now an adult who can and must communicate with her sister directly. While you can assist in the background, there no longer is a role for Mommy in resolving disputes.

*As a widow with grown children living on the West Coast, I find holidays like Mother's Day and Father's Day quite depressing. Any suggestions on how to cope with them?*

—Sad on Special Days,
Building 2

You are not alone in feeling depressed on these holidays, even if your children send cards and gifts to signify their appreciation of you. On other holidays, like Thanksgiving, or on religious holidays, it I more likely to be included by extended family and friends. But being alone when others are with their families makes it doubly hard on you.

Remembering these holidays when your children were young and your husband alive creates nostalgic thoughts that can be both negative and positive. The contrast of then and now could make you feel down, but on the other hand reliving the happy times can bring you some solace.

One way of coping with these holidays is to find other widows who are in a similar situation, with their children not available, and plan an interesting activity with them. This may mean going to a theater, a museum, or a movie. Going to a restaurant that caters to families on these holidays may make it more difficult for you, so go with friends to a diner or Chinese restaurant that is less family oriented.

The best solution is to plan on spending these holidays with your children if possible. Suggest visiting them to coincide with Mother's Day, or treat the family to a visit to you if that is feasible. This plan may be complicated for several reasons—see next question for more on that. Holiday expectations, with their social pressures, often create in us a range of emotions. Remember, the good news is that these holidays only come once a year.

———

*While I looked forward to spending every Mother's Day with my children and grand-children, in reality the planning has become a hassle, and the time together is always tense. Am I being ungrateful? How can I enjoy these special days?*
    —Wishing for Hassle-Free Holidays,
        Building 3

While we look forward to celebrating special days with our families, often we are disappointed because of unrealistic expectations. The ideal family, where everyone gets along and has similar needs, is a rarity, and issues always arise: What restaurant or home should we celebrate in? What time should we eat?

If you have several children, and they have in-laws living locally, there is always the issue of either including the in-laws in the plans to see you or choosing who sees whom and at what time. Some families may decide the daughter or son and some of the grandchildren should spend time with you, and the daughter-in-law or son-in-law and some grandchildren can spend time with the other parent/grandparent. While this plan has a downside, it also allows you time with your children without their spouses present. This hopefully encourages closeness without adult children having to make difficult choices.

The key to these holidays is flexibility and an awareness that others in the family are also struggling with the need to please many different people with varied expectations of what the holidays should be. You can enjoy this day by appreciating that some effort is being made to see you and bring you a gift. Overlook the fact that the teenage grandchildren seem bored or that someone had too much to drink.

Show gratitude for any gifts you get and try your best to avoid competitive feelings. Remember you are fortunate to have your family living nearby; those who have no family to celebrate with would indeed consider you ungrateful. Work at focusing on the positive of the situation rather than the negatives so you can enjoy the holiday.

—————

*Holiday time and holiday dinners are always stressful! My sister is constantly confiding in me about the details of her terrible marriage, and*

*when I act unloving and distant to my brother-in-law, she accuses me of being cold. It seems I am in a no-win situation. Any suggestions?*
                                    —Not So Merry,
                                    Building 2

You certainly are in a no-win situation that parallels taking sides in a marital separation or divorce. It is wonderful that you and your sister have a close relationship and that she is comfortable sharing her feelings with you. But knowing too much information about her marriage, particularly if they are staying together, is counterproductive to you and your relationship with your brother-in-law.

Since your sister uses you to vent and doesn't seem to be asking for advice, it is my suggestion that you tell her she can no longer complain about her husband to you. This seems like a chronic situation in which she feels better after the talk and you feel worse, with anger building up against her husband. They may make up after a fight and she only shares the negatives in the relationship with you. Even giving advice never works in such a situation, since you hear only one side of the story and are likely to take your sister's side.

The hard part will be for you to continue to be a caring and concerned sister and be strong in your resolution not to listen to her marital complaints.

———

*I feel foolish complaining, but I'm having dif-
ficulty dealing with the changes in my family.
Both of my adult children are married, and
holidays are not as they used to be. The children are either celebrating with their in-laws
or off on a vacation. I still celebrate with my
extended family, but it's not the same as the
good old days.*
                    —Remembering Christmases Past,
                                        Building 3

You seem to be aware that the big picture is positive,
in that both your children have moved on in their lives
and have partners. Yet your feelings of loss are understandable, since the definition of family involves your
children and memories of the past family celebrations.

Sharing your children with their spouses and in-
laws requires a generosity that is hard to muster when
you're feeling hurt. Of course you wish they would
choose to spend all holidays with you and your husband, but that is not realistic.

There are some solutions to this dilemma. The first
involves bringing the entire extended family together,
which is often a logistical problem if all children and
their spouses and in-laws are included. Sometimes

a restaurant or similar venue might be considered. The second and more practical solution is a planned alternating schedule of holiday celebrations that must be agreed upon by all who are involved. If the in-law family is of a different religion, it eliminates several holidays you are competing over. But Thanksgiving must be on a planned alternate schedule.

A more creative approach may be to redefine a Thanksgiving holiday if your children are not available to celebrate with you. This may mean a local getaway or a more elaborate vacation. If a new adventure doesn't help with your feelings of loss, it may be time for introspection! When children leave the nest and form families of their own, parents often have midlife crises. Involvement in a career, new activities, hobbies, volunteering, etc. may be a way of coming to terms with this new phase of your life.

It is also important not to compare yourself to others such as family and friends whose relationships with their adult children may be different from yours.

Try to take the lead from your children and not be too demanding of their time. Spend time with them in mutually enjoyed activities that are fun and stress-free.

The next phase of your life may include grand-parenting. This provides a different opportunity to interact with your children and their children. But again this time must be shared with the other set of grandparents, and you have to be aware of your potential for jealous feelings. It is important to be reasonable in your expectations and find joy and pleasure in these interactions.

Oh, the complexities of interpersonal relationships!

———

With summer soon upon us, I am looking forward to the impending weddings of several friends' children. Only months—or was it a year ago?—the sagas began, and I, as an empathetic listener, heard many of the details. Some were major issues, like interfaith couplings, and some were minor, like wedding venues, color schemes, and who is paying for what.

At times I inwardly lost patience with the friend to whom I was listening and would have liked to say that they should try not to lose sight of the bigger issue: that two young people who love each other are ready to make a commitment and take on the responsibilities of a life together. Marriage is difficult at best, and the problems of extended family expectations can pose additional burdens on the new couple. Of course, as a therapist, I also realized that some of what sounded trivial was only masking parental disappointments, hurts, and fears.

Trying to focus on the positive when friends are

negative is often trying. They don't want you to point out all the wonderful things you see. Usually they want validation that their perceptions are accurate, and they want your support for their position.

This basic approach to life may be characterized simply as a battle between the optimists and pessimists. Try as I did with one patient over several years, I came to realize she had a vested interest in believing that only bad things happened to her. She minimized anything positive and focused on the negatives in most of her relationships. It was as if she remained most comfortable in the role of victim.

I'd like to contrast this mode of adaptation with that of our dear friend and neighbor, Blossom Finehirsh, who passed away last month. While I did not know Blossom personally, all can remember her winning smile, her ever-present circle of friends, and her positive spirit despite her many struggles. The outpouring of love to her husband Rick attests to his continuing optimism and positive approach to life.

For more thoughts on a positive approach to life, I've consulted a book entitled *The Forgiving Self: The Road From Resentment to Connection* by Robert Karen, PhD. It was published in 2003 by Doubleday. Excerpts from the book intrigue me—most importantly that forgiveness is not a moral or religious issue, one of right and wrong. Instead forgiveness comes from understanding the complexities of life. In relationships most people share responsibility and blame, without one being the victim and the other the wrongdoer. People learn to tolerate ambiguity and ambivalence, and with maturity their grudges and festering resentments can be worked through. When anger is overwhelming, it takes its toll on the body, but most people have difficulty with unexpressed anger and with finding creative and connected ways to work out problems. As happened with my former patient, gnawing grudges take on their own lives.

Forgiveness must be genuine and from the heart. Otherwise, if you forgive because it seems expected of you, you will feel like a victim, and your resentments will grow.

*When it comes to buying gifts for my family for special occasions, I am so indecisive and troubled about whether they will like what I choose. Isn't this supposed to be a positive experience? Any suggestions?*
                    —Buyer's Remorse Blues,
                              Building 3

You are not alone with this dilemma. While giving a gift should be a heartwarming experience, it is often a complicated time for many of us. The traditions of one's family play an important part in how we approach gift-giving. In some families members like to be surprised, and in other families they prefer to give suggestions or even shop with you for the gift. Receiving a check or gift certificate is preferred by some while others like more personal gifts.

To complicate matters your children share your traditions, but their spouses' families may have very different approaches to gifts. It is important to learn about the receiver of the gift so you don't impose your values or have unrealistic expectations when you give a gift. For example, an expensive gift to your daughter-in-law may or may not be accepted graciously depending on attitudes. In contrast you may be disappointed when you receive only a card and a box of candy from her. You can choose to be hurt about this, or you can modify your giving in the future.

Gifts are only tokens that symbolize our love and caring and should not be attempts to buy affection or prove something. For some people giving takes on a competitive element. For example the other grandparents give a substantial monetary gift to your grandchild while you are unable to do the same. In this case a more personal gift, like something of your own or a day trip to the zoo or theater, would be equally appreciated.

Buying for someone who has everything or can afford most anything can also be problematic. Think creatively and offer some service like babysitting or home sitting, or treat them to a massage, a tennis lesson, or bridge lessons. Remember there is enough stress in life, so don't create more for yourself.

———

> *The wonderful news is my daughter is engaged and we are planning her wedding. However a complication has arisen concerning my ex-husband of twenty years. He has been in her life to some degree, but now he and my daughter's stepmother are making demands about wedding plans and their guest list. My daughter is very upset and doesn't even want him at the wedding, no less walking her down the aisle. I am not sure if or how I should intercede at this time.*
>
> —The Reluctant Mediator,
> Building 1

Congratulations on this happy event and the mixed blessing it has engendered. In the best of situations, planning for a wedding is stressful, usually because not everyone is in agreement about large and small details. There are usually just two families involved, but in cases of divorce a third family may make their demands too.

Without more information about the relationships

involved, it is difficult for me to advise you. It seems most important that you keep lines of communication open with your daughter, who seems very angry with her father. Obviously her relationship with her father over the past twenty years must be considered; i.e., has he provided financial support? Has he spent quality time with her? Your relationship with your ex is important as well. I hope that you encouraged your daughter to see her father regardless of whether he provided support, and that you did not criticize him or his wife.

I am inferring you are unsure if you have a role as mediator at this time. You don't want to become estranged from your daughter, but you are concerned about the long-term effect on the father-daughter relationship if you don't intervene. You seem aware that your daughter may be overreacting and that she may later regret a decision she makes now about her father's participation in her wedding.

I suggest you share with your daughter the dilemma you are experiencing. Also you can have her discuss the situation with others she respects, like her aunt or sister, if you or she feels you can't be objective. If you feel she is responsive, you can make suggestions that give her additional options she might not be able to consider at present. You can, with her permission, speak to her father if she is unable to do so once a solution is reached.

Your daughter's fiancé may be another resource

in helping her think through the situation in a less emotional way. I would hope that such an important milestone like marriage would not be characterized by animosity, and that all family members can put aside their differences and enjoy this joyful event. One should worry that they would look back and regret the impulsive actions taken in the past.

I believe you should try to help your daughter at this time in a sensitive and careful way. It is part of motherhood to guide our children even when they are young adults.

———

*We have been invited to the wedding of a great-niece whom we haven't seen in many years. Our niece has not been in contact with us despite overtures on my part to keep in touch. Her mother—my sister-in-law—does speak to us several times a year, but obviously the relationship is not close. I feel uncomfortable about this invitation and wonder if they are just looking for a gift. What's your take on this?*

—Not-Feeling-So-Great Aunt,
Building 2

It seems clear that you are hurt about the lack of contact these last years from family you may have been close with at one time. Friendships continue through ongoing communication, yet families remain families despite the lack of what we consider an ongoing relationship. The invitation may be more of an obligation toward family than a genuine wish to have you be a part of a *simcha*.

Just think how you would feel if you did not receive an invitation! The family estrangement would be a permanent one. You now have an opportunity to rebuild a relationship with your niece if you so desire. I doubt the family is just inviting you for a gift, especially with what weddings cost today. This seems like a reaching out that you can accept or reject. Why not be gracious and accept, since family ties can prove meaningful?

*My daughter, who is engaged to be married soon, has been complaining about her mother-in-law to be, who she perceives as being intrusive, especially now during the wedding preparations. She has asked for my help, and I'm not sure how to advise her. Any suggestions?*
—Befuddled Mother of the Bride,
Building 2

I suggest you help her focus on the positives and not point out negative traits you might also see. Most important is the fact the mother-in-law reared a young man whom your daughter loves and wants to spend her life with. Yet it is important that your daughter feels supported by you during this tense time and that she has a person who can listen to her gripes. You can empathize with her without actually agreeing with her.

It is critical that she be discrete in discussing these concerns with her fiancé, even if he voices similar problems with his mother. This is the start of a new family constellation, and something said can come back to haunt her in the future. No son should be put into the middle of a conflicted relationship between his wife and his mother.

While it may seem disingenuous, advise your daughter to be pleasant and respectful when spending time with her mother-in-law. This does not mean she can't set some rules and boundaries with the cooperation of her husband, such as convenient times for telephone calls, calling before visiting, how often you have dinner together, and how holiday meals might be spent. These discussions are best held after the wedding, when setting up the new home.

When dealing with wedding plan decisions, a time that is generally fraught with conflicts because of different needs and values, your daughter can be somewhat evasive. She can say she will check with her parents, and she can ask you and your husband to intercede, which will protect her. You can be the heavy if need be!

Lastly you have served as a role model with your own mother-in-law. Hopefully you have worked out a successful relationship; if not you can point out what hasn't worked and what you have learned. Wisdom comes with experience.

# Parenting:
# The Adventure of a Lifetime

Motherhood is a full-time job when your children are small, and it turns into a lifetime commitment. The recent news story out of Nebraska about parents surrendering their older children to state custody under the Safe Haven Law calls to our attention the struggles that are often part of being a parent.

Coincidentally, within the last few weeks, several friends have shared their frustration with me over their roles in the mothering experience with their adult children. We discussed issues arising from health and employment. In three cases adult daughters told their parents about serious medical problems but did not ask for advice or assistance in finding doctors or hospitals that specialize in the illnesses. The moms remain worried and feel, rightfully so, that they cannot gain any control in these situations.

Most of us, when faced with crises, plan coping strategies or courses of action that help us cope with our feelings. Such plans are excellent survival strategies.

But what can we do when crises affect our children? While your children do know you love them and want the best for them, tell them you understand their fears and are willing to respect their needs to handle matters without your help. Using humor by saying mothers are supposed to worry may open up communication.

An indirect tactic might be to offer the name of someone who has a similar health problem. This may give your child the necessary distance from you and may allow him or her to receive necessary information from a surrogate. However this surrogate must offer confidentiality about the discussion if that's what your child wants. While this takes you out of the loop, you may be less anxious knowing someone else is serving as an advisor.

Children of all ages need to feel autonomous, and they often bristle at receiving unsolicited advice. The alternative is having a very dependent child who is incapable of making decisions and assuming full responsibility in his or her life.

Other friends have shared with me stories of children who have lost jobs and won't discuss their plans in any way. As parents you can feel useful by offering some temporary financial help. Yet don't expect your child also to take advice about employment, even though this may frustrate you and lead to anger about your inability to be heard, considering your years of experience.

Again, in such a situation, the autonomy of the adult child is clearly being threatened. The loss of a job affects self-esteem, and with that the child's defenses rise. There is a tendency to withdraw and show a façade of confidence in the face of shame and humiliation. A parent must be a cheerleader, supporting the child from the sidelines and content with a minimal role. Most children realize their parents' help—known as unconditional love—is available should they want advice.

The plight of the parents in these scenarios is common. One must learn that bearing the anxiety and fear of the ill child or the anger and frustration of the child who is unwilling to interact in the fashion of the family on the TV show *Father Knows Best* is a realistic dilemma.

*While Mother's Day was a wonderful opportunity to be with my children, their spouses, and my grandchildren, I am upset about the way my daughter-in-law feeds her children. I feel like saying something to her, but I don't know how to go about it without hurting her feelings. What do you advise?*
—Good Nutrition Grandma,
Building 2

The problem of dealing with your daughter-in- law is a complex one, but the solution is simple. I'll quote from a new book by Jane Isay, entitled *Walking on Eggshells—Navigating the Delicate Relationship Between Adult Children and Parents*. Isay states a long overdue eleventh commandment: "thou shalt not give your grown children advice."

This adage, however, is not always easy to follow. Adult children often maintain close ties with their parents, especially if they need economic or emotional support. Generous parents often have strings attached to their giving, and both parties may have ambivalent feelings about this type of relationship.

To complicate matters, the mother-in-law and daughter-in-law relationship is fraught with even more complexities. And you are placing your son in a difficult position if you choose to say anything that is clearly negative to his wife. Unless there is imminent danger to your grandchildren, your parenting suggestions will not be welcomed, and you will be perceived as interfering and critical.

It is the rare adult child who will ask his or her parents for advice on raising kids. If he or she does ask, you can give your opinion, but be aware of overstepping your bounds. Motherhood never ends, but a positive relationship with adult children requires a high level of diplomacy!

*I am concerned about my thirty-five-year-old granddaughter. While she lives on her own, she spends most weekends with her parents, my son and daughter-in-law. She goes to the gym with her folks, takes golf or tennis lessons at their club, and goes to the movies and dinner with them. She often takes vacations with them too. I think this is unnatural but wonder if I should say anything.*

Concerned,

Building 1

I understand your concern in hoping that your granddaughter meets an appropriate mate and eventually marries. It may be that she currently has few single friends and is lonely. Her parents are caring and able to provide exciting and fun weekends for her, but unless there are opportunities at the club to meet contemporaries she is not enlarging her social network. Your role in this is limited because interference would not be welcome by your granddaughter or her parents.

If you are close to your granddaughter, invite her to lunch and offer her a gift of a week at golf or tennis camp with her peers, or a trip geared toward her age group. Bring some brochures from a travel agent, which would show you have put some thought into this. While there is no guaranteed she will not be angry with you, this might open up a discussion. Perhaps her single friends are all in group-share houses in the Hamptons or on Fire Island, and she either hates that scene or can't afford it. You can offer monetary assistance if that is holding her back. Most important is the relationship you are developing with this young lady, who may not be as comfortable telling her parents how much time she wants to spend with them.

*I'm a grandmother of two school-aged children who live a half hour away. I cared for the youngest when my daughter was working and am very close to the children. However, when I call and want to visit, my daughter puts me off and makes me feel that I am being intrusive. I feel hurt and don't know what to do. Any suggestions?*

*—Meddling Mama,*
*Building 3*

It's understandable that you're hurt and feel rejected, especially since you were the caretaker of your youngest grandchild some years ago. Your relationship then was co-parent, and your closeness grew as a result to this time you spent with the child. You may feel exploited because you expected more appreciation from your daughter. Rather than receiving the kudos you want, you are made to feel guilty for calling and wanting to visit.

This dilemma requires great sensitivity on your part. If you express your feelings truthfully, your daughter may get very defensive and pull away more. I feel it is better to state that you miss the children and would like to plan on seeing them for dinner, with or without the parents, once a week. You can name a weekday night and offer to meet the children after school. Or ask your daughter to choose the night so it doesn't interfere with the children's extracurricular activities. Your daughter and her husband might enjoy a midweek date when you are with the children.

The "plan ahead" idea takes some pressure off both of you. Telephone calls also might be prearranged. Asking your daughter when the best time to call is advisable, since a working mother is beset with dinner, homework help, etc. What you perceive as rejection when you call may be irritation due to bad timing, and because she may not yet know her weekend schedule and if the children has time for a visit. Try to be sympathetic to your daughter although you feel angry. Ask her if there is something you can do to help her, like shopping or bringing over a meal.

Spending quality time with the grandchildren

is wonderful and makes them feel special and loved. The time you gave in caring for them in the past was significant, and don't forget that you gained something from that time as well. You may not have the physical closeness you once had with the children, but perhaps you can direct your need to nurture others to pets or volunteer work with children or seniors, rather than focusing exclusively on the grandchildren.

———

*I have a wonderful and successful forty-five-year-old daughter who I consider a best friend. Yet when we see each other, there is often tension in the air. Recently I commented on her hair, and she overreacted and told me to stop criticizing her. I don't understand, since I was only being honest. Can you explain?*

—Blunt Betty,
Building 2

———

As I discussed in my column last month, relationships with adult children are quite complex, and mother-daughter interactions are markedly difficult.

Deborah Tannen, a professor of linguistics at Georgetown University, wrote a book called *You're Wearing THAT? Understanding Mothers and Daughters in Conversation* (2006). Her findings were based on five years of research in which she analyzed taped conversations between mothers and daughters.

The mother-daughter relationship reflects an ongoing search for the right balance of closeness and distance, and characterizing the relationship as "friends" underestimates the power a mother still may possess.

A comment by a friend does not have the same meaning as something said by a mother. Remarks about the daughter's hair, clothing, and weight are particularly touchy! Tannen found that any comment, suggestion, or offer of help by a loving and caring mother may be interpreted as a criticism by the daughter.

Don't forget that adult children still want the unconditional love and approval of their parents, even though they intellectually understand their mothers may not like everything they do. Even when your daughter asks for advice, be cautious of what you say, since misinterpretations are likely. Your daughter may really want your blessing and not your honest opinion.

A relationship where confidences are shared implies a closeness that is positive, but there are risks involved as well. In such situations it is more difficult to hide imperfections and not be scrutinized. It is a rare mother who can be nonjudgmental when offering advice.

Tannen said mothers complain that they can't open their mouths because their daughters take everything as criticisms. When a daughter asks if her new outfit is slimming, or how you like her haircut, beware that you may be stepping into a trap. Be positive and generous with your praise. Otherwise you may have to contend with anger and retaliation from your daughter, as you did. You will end up feeling hurt and shut out, and your relationship may suffer over the short and long haul.

The scenario you presented is not uncommon and does not reflect a fatally flawed relationship. But be aware that the truth can be hurtful and may put your relationship in jeopardy!

———

*I have five grandchildren, and I have a special relationship with the oldest, who is twenty-six. At times she asks me if she is my favorite. I handle it by saying, "You're my favorite green-eyed grandchild," since she is the only green-eyed one. Am I handling this correctly?*
*—Playing Favorites,*
*Building 1*

The wonderful part of your question is the fact that there is closeness with this twenty-plus young lady, who generally is involved with other parts of her life now. This bond is probably based on the love and affection you gave this first grandchild, who may also have lived nearby. She may experience this specialness you describe, and she should feel comfortable in this knowledge.

It is not clear why she asked if she is the favorite at this time. It could be a joking interplay you've had for years, or perhaps it's a response to something that just occurred. If great attention is being given to her sibling who graduated with honors, for example, she could be jealous of this other grandchild. Issues of competition arise all the time, so be aware of what may be motivating her question. Your granddaughter may be feeling insecure now because of some setback in her life, and she may require some extra reassurance at this time. Try to be available and loving, but also look for what makes each grandchild special and unique. You don't want to be accused of playing favorites.

*At a holiday dinner for twenty-five at my daughter's house, I was concerned about my two grandsons playing computer games at the table. They ate little and did not engage*

*in conversation with anyone. Their parents
said there was nothing they could do about
the situation. I am distressed about the lack
of parental responsibility in teaching their
children manners. This extends to acknowledging gifts as well.*
      —Old-Fashioned Grandma,
               Building 1

Your letter strikes a note with many grandparents
I spoke to. Yet the solution to such a situation is very
complex and may be dependent upon the existing
relationship with your children and grandchildren.
While the age of your grandsons was not mentioned
in the letter, this problem extends to young adults too
who are busy texting, involved with their phones and
BlackBerrys. It appears that even adults may not be
courteous in this new ear of electronic communication.

Firstly a large family gathering is not the time to
reprimand your grandchildren or criticize their parents in front of an audience. Sometimes a humorous
comment about the Stone Age, when you didn't have
such diversions, might have some effect and might
initiate some conversation.

If a grandson is sitting next to you, you might
quietly share your disappointment and say you were
hoping to hear about school, their sports teams, or

some hobby. If you're helping in the kitchen, you might tell your daughter about your concerns and she might discretely ask her sons to put away their computer games. However your letter seems to indicate that she may not feel it is inappropriate for them to be playing at the table. Then it is difficult to impose your values on the family.

The age of the grandchildren is relevant, I think. If the boys are young, under ten or so, it may be difficult for them to remain at the table without being disruptive. In such a case, they might be excused after a period to watch TV, especially if the dinner is at their home.

Before the next get-together, whether it's a small birthday dinner at a restaurant or a larger gathering, try to encourage your daughter to set some rules about electronics, which also can apply to adults and their cell phones.

Building relationships with your grandchildren is important, and you might make individual dates with them for a swim, lunch, or a movie. In this way you'll have opportunities to influence them directly. In a nonjudgmental way you could let them know you were disappointed at the dinner that they were not participating. Using "I" statements makes others less defensive and opens lines of communication.

It is hard to counteract your children's child-rearing

practices. Again, saying you were hurt that the boys didn't call to thank you for the Chanukah gifts is better than using terms like "rude." Try to teach by setting an example. Sending your daughter a thank-you note after the holiday dinner is a start.

While your anger and frustration over events at the holiday dinner may be justified, perhaps you can try to reframe, or look at the evening in a different way. You are fortunate to have family nearby who include you in holiday festivities. Sometimes it's difficult to see the bright side of the situation!

———

*As a grandmother and former teacher, I am concerned about my twelve-year-old grandson, who is doing poorly in school and is beginning to act out physically to avoid school. My son and daughter-in-law are minimizing the problem. What can I do to help my grandson and deal with his parents?*
—An Education Advocate,
Building 2

You have to be concerned about being the intrusive mother and mother-in-law even though you have serious concerns about your grandson and his health and welfare.

Depending upon your relationship with your grandson, you can first be available to talk with him and offer some tutoring help at homework time. You can begin to judge how he is coping with the situation and how open he is about what's transpiring. Teenage years are difficult, and hopefully he is able to talk to you more easily than his parents, who he is concerned about disappointing. If he has a successful older sibling, this makes it harder for him.

You can discretely begin a conversation with the parents around report card time by asking what the teachers and guidance counselor have said and suggested. His parents might be reluctant to have school personnel conduct a formal evaluation to detect whether there is a learning disability, which in turn can create emotional problems. This is where you might step in and offer to pay for a private evaluation by a psychologist.

It is very important that you be supportive and not judgmental about their reluctance to acknowledge a problem. Be empathetic about their concerns for privacy if that's an issue. Most important point out that your grandson's problem is not a reflection on them, and that if he had and illness like diabetes you know they would get him the proper help. You're in a difficult position, but persist for your grandson's sake.

⪘

*I recently spent time with my grown children and found we have strained relationships with little to talk about, especially if I want to keep the peace. I feel frustrated and disappointed. Is this normal? What can I do to improve matters?*
                    —Tired of Talking to Myself,
                              Building 1

While this may not be the normal situation, it is quite common. If other parents were open about their family relationships, you would feel better knowing all is not perfect in other households. Instead you may hear friends lauding their children and their accomplishments, and you feel badly that your family does not measure up.

However, in close relationships with friends you're more likely to have honest discussions about their children and the day-to-day conflicts that create frustration. Sometimes these situations are transitory, and other times they are chronic. The situations may vary depending on whether the children live nearby or out of town. Divorce of having special-needs children complicate relationships even further.

There are generally common issues in parent-child

relationships. Briefly, as a parent you feel you loved and nurtured your children and gave them the best you could. As a mother you may have devoted yourself to their care and defined yourself in this role. You received the satisfaction that you were doing a good job because of the closeness and love they gave back to you.

Then comes adolescence, when it's healthy for children to pull away and begin to assert their independence. At this time parents can do nothing right—they are often criticized and rejected by their teenagers so a comfortable distance is attained. As a parent it's difficult to remain loving and accepting when faced with this negative behavior. Most parent-child relationships move beyond this open warfare, sometimes with time and maturity, and other times with professional help like family counseling.

Yet even after many years these conflicts can reemerge. A simple statement by you may be construed as a criticism by an insecure adult child. Your child's inability to go with you to the doctor is experienced as unloving and uncaring by you. How do we begin to feel less vulnerable in these relationships? How do we move ahead and repair the parent-child bond?

The strain you experienced when you saw your children may reflect that there are issues that are left unsaid. It is difficult at best to have an intimate discussion about feelings. Certainly one-to-one time with a child provides an opportunity to broach topics that are hard to discuss. It's important to take responsibility for the part you play in the relationship rather than making your child feel guilty and defensive. If you start by sharing your feelings and saying, "I feel bad that we aren't as close as we were," it can create a tense situation. Most of us are not comfortable with or experienced in sharing our feelings even in the most intimate relationships.

Often we show feelings through our actions rather than with words. We may offer to babysit, invite the children to dinner, and buy gifts as ways to express our positive feelings. On the other hand, if we are angry we may do the opposite by turning down invitations, being critical, or just being remote and distant. It's difficult to be loving and accepting when you feel hurt or rejected. Remember your child's adolescence!

There is certainly a risk in beginning open communication with your child, but the reward is great when issues can be put to rest. Depending on your level of comfort, you can take a tentative step toward opening communication. You may not be effective in turning a troubled relationship around, but at least you can take comfort in knowing you have tried to bridge the gap.

*As a stepmother of two teenagers who visit on alternate weekends, I have heard complaints from their mother about their discomfort when visiting. I am very hurt by this since I go out of my way to entertain them and make them feel comfortable. Any suggestions?*
—Hostess With the Mostess—Or So I
Thought,
Building 3

Stepparent relationships at any age are tricky, and particularly with teenagers, who would prefer to spend time with their friends at home and participate in their usual activities instead of visiting. While their relationships with you might have been cordial when they were younger, as teenagers they are experiencing some independence and the beginnings of rebellious behavior, thus they are complaining more now.

It's unfortunate you heard this complaint from their mother and not your husband, since your relationship with their mother might be wrought with hostility and competitiveness, leaving you to question the validity of the situation. It would have been preferable if the children or their mother spoke to your husband about the issue so the two of you could discuss the visitation plans.

It's understandable that you're hurt by this, but

rather than be furious, become curious and try not to personalize this situation as an affront to you. You and your husband need to hear the specifics from the children themselves, since they are old enough to discuss their complaints. If they feel more comfortable talking just to their father, don't get defensive about that. As the children's needs change, there may have to be changes and accommodations in their visits, as well as activities planned.

Remember you are not their second mother but should serve as a loving friend to your stepchildren. That is a very difficult role to fill.

*I have been married for twenty-two years. Both my husband and I have adult married children from our first marriages. The relationships with our stepchildren are cordial but tense most of the time. This is particularly noticeable during holiday dinners, when all our children are together. It is also obvious when we go out with each other's children. Any suggestions to smooth the way?*
                          *—Stuck in a Stoic Stepfamily,*
                                        *Building 3*

Wouldn't it be wonderful if holidays were like old-time Hollywood movies? After twenty-two years of marriage and life with stepchildren, I would reconcile myself to the fact that there may not be a significant change in your family dynamics. You surely worked on this relationship through the years, serving as a concerned friend rather than a replacement parent.

Rather than everyone being comfortable when both families are together, you might consider an alternative plan and occasionally celebrate separately. You might extend this plan for informal get-togethers where you spend time with your children without your husband, and he does similarly. This may be a rather simple way to diminish the tension and in turn eliminate marital discord as it relates to the children.

This revolutionary idea of having separate activities, including time alone with your children, may redefine your marital contract. I think of marriages as dependent, interdependent, or independent relationships. For some couples a good relationship is defined by the fact that they do everything together. Others, however, feel very comfortable with their separate activities, but dinners out and visits with children have always been together activities.

I am suggesting that this pattern be reconsidered. You might discuss this with your stepchildren so they don't feel rejected or hurt by the change. Alone time is a positive dimension and can enhance your marriage as well as reduce the stress of dealing with the stepchildren, who you might appreciate more when getting together is of your choosing rather than mandatory.

———

*My sister and I have grown distant since we disagreed two years ago about our mother's possible move to an assisted living facility. Mom asked me to intervene and persuade my sister that she could remain at home, and Mom stayed home. After a recent fall, she is now in a facility, but my sister still holds a grudge over my role two years ago. What can I do to repair our relationship?*

—On Mom's Side,
Building 1

I suggest you take your sister to lunch to begin to repair your relationship. It appears that your mother may have manipulated you two years ago without your being fully aware of it or understanding your mom's health status. Your mom, with her failing health, must have felt out of control and thus used you in her conflict with your sister over her move.

When you were children, your sister may have played these same games by complaining about you and getting your mother to take sides. This strategy is common when you feel powerless. I think it's best if you apologize to your sister and point out how you didn't give enough credence to her assessment of your mom's health then. (You may have inferred less noble motivation on your sister's part.) Also point out that you were manipulated into taking Mom's side without understanding all the implications, perhaps while trying to gain recognition as the "good" daughter.

Promise to work together in the future as a cooperative team when deciding matters concerning your mom.

# Happiness

A t the start of the New Year, we make our annual resolutions, which are generally specific to a material want or need. We often wish for good health and aspire to vague notions of happiness without thinking about how we can achieve these illusive goals.

In the November 9, 2004 edition of *Family Circle*, an article entitled "The Simple Secrets of Happiness" caught my attention. I'd like to share some points made by the author, Glenn Paskin, based upon his interviews with Deepak Chopra, MD, and Anthony Robbins—both experts on human growth and development.

Both Chopra and Robbins equate happiness with a more fulfilling life, which is a very personal challenge for all of us. They believe the capacity to grow and evolve continues throughout life and is characterized by remaining curious and mentally, emotionally, and physically engaged.

It sounds easy, but it takes effort to push or stretch ourselves. We often play it safe and stay with familiar routines rather than risk taking chances. By being over-cautious we inhibit our growth and limit our chances for happiness. We also forget to have fun, and we don't understand that playfulness increases creativity and leads to growth and happiness.

The article mentioned two factors that interfere with growth. The first is our tendency to falsely believe that material things can buy happiness rather than understanding that happiness is part of an internal process. The second factor is our tendency to focus on the negative aspects of our lives and not maturely move ahead.

Chopra and Robbins suggest you question yourself and ask what need is not being met when you experience unhappiness. While this is not an easy task, it may help you focus on whether your relationships and your physical, spiritual, or intellectual being are affected. In this way you can try to solve the problem that is thwarting your happiness and growth.

There are several ways to attempt to achieve your goals. By assuming the mindset of a child, you can begin to see things with hopeful and fresh eyes and explore the world in a new way. By embracing change and giving up the tedium of your life, you will have the opportunity to be inspired and challenged to grow, and a sense of wonder will return to you. Chopra and Robbins both mention how physical activity, a creative hobby, or laughter can enhance your mood. Lastly they focus on the human capacity to love as well as our ability to care for and help others. In giving to others you also give to yourself, and it is through this form of love that you can grow spiritually.

This article presents a challenge to take responsibility for our own happiness.

During my winter stay in Florida, I had time to read an interesting article that has relevance to our everyday lives and our relationships with others. It responds to the proverbial question of why one feels discontent much of the time, even when on the surface things seem to be going well.

The article, entitled "The Tyranny of Choice," was written by Barry Schwartz and appeared in the *Scientific American* of April 2004. It detailed studies by various social scientists. Its basic premise was that while the opportunity to make choices enhances our lives, more choices are not always better than fewer choices.

There are theories about why some people end up unhappy rather than pleased when their options increase. People called *maximizers* strive to check out every option, and these people are the least happy with the fruits of their efforts, as compared with *satisfiers* who aim for good enough. The satisfiers are happier, more optimistic, and less depressed, and don't tend to brood or ruminate once they make decisions.

When a selection is chosen, there is the cost of losing the opportunity a different option would have afforded. In addition people may also suffer regret about the options they settle on, and this regret can lead to dissatisfaction and even possibly to depression. Regret about what we did not choose and disappointment with what we did choose affects many of us, even if the final decisions were not bad. One example is spending four months deciding on what computer to buy or where to go on vacation, only to find that you are excited or pleased for only a short time.

Because of the principle called *adaptation*, enthusiasm about positive experiences does not sustain itself. Dr. D. Gilbert and Dr. T. Wilson of the University of Virginia have shown that people consistently mispredict how long good experiences will make them feel good and how long bad experiences will make them feel bad. This waning of pleasure comes as an unpleasant surprise and causes more disappointment in a world of many options than in a world of few options.

The amount of choice in most aspects of our lives corresponds to the raising of expectations, and in turn this may cause us distress. While having choices has a positive effect on us, psychological benefits start to level off and can lead to choice-related distress.

It is important to recognize and take steps to reduce the negative effects of numerous choices in decision making. Some options to consider are:

- Choose when to choose.
- Learn to accept good enough.
- Don't worry about what you're missing.
- Control your expectations.

# Dating, Mating, and Relating

North Shore Towers is unique in its residents' abilities to support those who are coping with loneliness after becoming widows or widowers. While one tends initially to retreat and want to be left alone, experience shows that moving toward others for lunch, dinner, card games, or movies can begin to relieve some of the sadness and anxiety that is experienced after losing a spouse.

While I haven't read the book *Epilogue*, a review in *The New York Times* on August 24, 2008 described this new book, written by well-known author Anne Roiphe, whose husband died in December 2005. Her goal was to present a bereaved person's efforts to restore the rhythms of a normal existence.

In her book Roiphe admits being alone and mourning a long-term mate is not easily resolved. She quotes an essay by psychoanalyst Frieda Fromm Reichmann, called "Loneliness": "Loneliness presents a threat to a person's integrity and well-being, to the very sense of who one is... Loneliness is so awful an experience that most people will do anything to avoid it."

In addition to loneliness, Roiphe experienced vague anxiety about nothing in particular, with no sense to it, and it flowed in and out of her mind all day.

With time, as days and months passed, the worst symptoms of her shock and panic receded, as did her insomnia. She even began to feel moments of joy when with her daughters and their families. This love of family seemed to banish her numbness, fragility, and fear. It was hard to avoid the trap of self-pity, and she longingly thought of happier times. After that phase she decided simply to go forward and keep going on despite her sadness.

No one can diminish the loss of a partner and soul mate, but you are not alone, and others can help you during this difficult time if you reach out.

*What is your advice regarding infidelity? Specifically, my cousin and his wife are good social friends who my husband and I see once a month. The wife asked me recently if her husband was having an affair, and I didn't know what to say. The truth is I have seen*

*him out with someone else, but I wonder if*
*honesty is called for in this situation.*
                              —Seen Too Much,
                                 Building 1

This is a tough call and would probably generate
a very heated discussion if posed to any group. In my
opinion I would think through the benefits and pitfalls
of telling her the truth. This is complicated by the fact
that the husband is your cousin. You will be perceived
as the bad guy if the marriage breaks up on the basis
of your information. Even if this couple stays together,
your knowing about the infidelity might become a sore
point and may lead to an estrangement between you
and the couple.

I also wonder if you believe that being asked point-
blank about the alleged infidelity is different from your
not telling her when you first suspected your cousin
was cheating. Obviously it is harder to lie when asked
than it was to share your suspicions when you saw him
out with someone.

We tell white lies all the time to protect hurting
people we care about. However this situation is more
serious than lying about liking a friend's haircut, new
couch, or new son-in-law; it has consequences that are
more far-reaching.

Two suggestions come to mind that take a middle

road. You might ask the wife why she thinks her husband is unfaithful, and you could suggest she pursue it directly with him, or perhaps hire a private detective to investigate. You might also speak to the husband—your cousin—privately and tell him his wife has asked you about his faithfulness. Depending on his response, you can decide if you want to share your suspicions with him. In this way you may be more helpful in saving this marriage.

---

*As a widow for eight months, I have been participating in a bereavement group for the last six months. Surprisingly a fellow support group member, a recent widower, and I developed a relationship, and we go out to dinner regularly. We are becoming emotionally involved with each other, and I feel like a teenager in love. However I am close with my two adult children and wonder if I should discuss this man and relationship with them.*
　　　　　　　—Falling for a New Friend,
　　　　　　　　　　Building 1

It is understandable that you want to share your joy with your children at this time, but I caution you that it may not be a wise decision to do so yet. While your children may be intellectually pleased that you are moving beyond your grief, emotionally they are probably not ready to think of you in a new relationship. Their ties to their father may be strong, and they may still be mourning his death. To introduce a new person into your family seems premature on several levels. You should be sensitive to your children's feelings too.

First of all you and your widower friend have not known each other very long, and it can be damaging to involve your children in the early stages of this new relationship. With both young children and adult children, rivalries and other issues can emerge that can negatively impact all of you. Your children's readiness can be discerned by dropping hints, talking about "a friend," or directly asking how they would feel if you started dating. It is most important that the meeting of your children and beau goes well if you want them to accept him and for the relationship to flourish.

Because the first year after a death is a very trying time for all, it is better to be cautious in this new relationship and not rush ahead. Follow your heart, but use your head.

———

*I have been living at NST for three years, since my divorce. My ex-wife recently sold her home and has just bought an apartment here*

*in another building. I am concerned about
how her move to the Towers will impact my
life. Any suggestions?*
—Bye Bye Privacy,
Building 3

Without knowing more about the quality of your relationship with your ex-wife, it is difficult to advise you. If you have co-parented your children or have adult children, it is reasonable to expect that you see each other regularly at family functions. Of course it will be more difficult to be civil to each other if you both carry grudges. Now may be the time to bury the hatchet—you did love this woman once.

The extent of your contact with your ex-wife will depend on what activities you are involved in at the Towers and whether you have mutual friends. You can try to avoid her if you are uncomfortable, but it seems more mature to treat her like an old friend and introduce her to your neighbors.

It is also unclear if either of you is involved in another relationship and how comfortable you will be with seeing her with another man, or with your being with another woman in her presence. In this world of complex dating scenarios, especially at the Towers, where dating couples have uncoupled, it seems best to be discrete in not discussing the ex with others.

Hopefully your ex-wife's move to the Towers will not have a negative impact on your life. It's up to you to find the positives in the situation—visits by your children and grandchildren will be easier, for example. Each of you may find a new love in the future, and you may both be able to move on and find happiness.

———

*I need advice on how to tell my two twen-tysomething sons that I am planning to remarry. Their mother and I separated a year and a half ago, and for a year I have been dating a wonderful woman who is my con-temporary. Both sons live out of town, and only one has met my intended.*
                      —Can't Keep It Secret,
                                Building 3

The good news is that you have met someone whose life you will share and who hopefully brings you happiness. Also the fact that your fiancée is your contemporary is in your favor. Imagine having to introduce your children to an intended who is their age or younger.

While I should not generalize, sons might have an easier time accepting a stepmother because their identification with their mother is usually not as strong as a daughter's is. However the circumstances of the divorce and their relationships with their mother plays a part in the family dynamics, and this should be considered. If their mother is also dating, this might make it easier for them to accept your significant other.

Specific advice would include a face-to-face dinner alone with your sons. Rather than mention an engagement that has already occurred, just talk about plans to get married and your excitement and joy about your intended. Express your hope that they will get to know her and accept her as a new member of the family. It is important to include them in forthcoming wedding plans and, especially since you live out of town, confer with them about convenient dates if you are planning a ceremony and/or reception. After this talk plan another get-together, perhaps in a restaurant, where your sons and your fiancée can meet. Depending on their initial reactions to the news, it might be best if the evening is structured and brief. Don't be disappointed if your sons are less than enthusiastic. It will take some time for them to get used to this new family constellation, but hopefully over time they will come to love and appreciate your new wife.

---

*We've been married for forty-two years, and I am recently retired while my husband still works. We recently moved to North Shore Towers, and I have made some good friends, some of whom are widows. My dilemma involves convincing my husband that I still love him when I choose to spend time playing cards or going shopping with friends. He feels that daytime activities with the women are fine, but he resents my spending any evenings away from him. I can't even bring up the idea of joining them for a weeklong elder hostel trip. Any suggestions?*

—Social Butterfly,
Building 2

There have been many recent changes in your life—retirement, new home, etc. You are fortunate to have met friends and have many activities to fill your leisure time. It is understandable that your husband is anxious about new routines. It may take some time for him to adjust to this situation, particularly if your marriage is defined by the togetherness I described in my previous response.

Does your husband have hobbies and activities he has not pursued in a while? If so encourage him to pursue them now so he can have something to occupy him in your absence. But don't be surprised or resentful if he begins to spend evenings without you. At North Shore Towers, he can meet new friends in the gym, card room, and golf club and have opportunities to prepare for his own retirement.

At the heart of your question is how to convince your husband that you still love him even if you spend time away from him. The quality of your relationship should not diminish by this new separateness. In fact the time you spend together may be valued more, and you'll have more to share about your activities and friends

Honestly communicate with him about your concern for him, and reassure him that he and your marriage are very important to you. . I might wait a while before taking a weeklong trip unless your husband has put off a fishing or ski trip because you were not interested in joining him. While you don't need his permission to take such a trip with friends, your sensitivity to his needs will be appreciated. There will be other opportunities for trips. Your need to fill your days may also reflect your anxiety about retirement, so go slowly.

———

*I'm a recent widower living at North Shore Towers, and I am interested in dating a neighbor. My children know of my intentions and are not in favor of this. Any suggestions?*
                                        —Ready to Jump In,
                                                    Building 2

It is a little late for my first suggestion, which would be not to tell your children of this plan. You may be close to your children, and you may confide in them, particularly at this time when you are lonely. However they may look at your dating someone as disrespectful to their late mother, and they may not be ready to include someone new in the family.

Since you didn't say how long you have been widowed, it is difficult to give advice. Within the first six to nine months, it is preferable to join a bereavement group where you can talk about your loss and feelings. Often members of such groups spend time outside meetings going to dinner or doing activities together as a means of coping with loneliness. You can also spend time with male friends or couples who will be able to provide some support. In addition it is important to develop new interests and hobbies. Senior centers and adult education programs offer such options.

It is important to feel ready for a new relationship after working through your grief and feelings, so the ghost of your wife doesn't intrude. Once you're at that point, you can spend time with your neighbor without discussing it with family and friends. Until you know if the relationship is serious, it is best to keep a low profile. (See the next question.) That means leaving the complex for dinner and movies and not introducing her to friends at first. You might find that you want to date more than one woman, and your family needs not be part of your new bachelor years.

———

*As a widow of five years, I have met a wonderful man at North Shore Towers who is interested in pursuing a relationship. I am concerned about our privacy and our neighbors knowing our business. Is it a good idea to date a neighbor?*
                              —Too Close for Comfort,
                                          Building 1

What a loaded question you pose. There are many factors to consider, and no one answer is right for everyone. North Shore Towers has been the meeting place of many couples, some of whom have gone on to wed. There are many single people living at the Towers, and there are many opportunities for them to meet when sharing interests and activities. Having friends in common also allows for introductions to be made.

Obviously there are conveniences when dating someone in the complex, but your privacy will certainly be compromised. Neighbors will see you together and will talk about it, but hopefully they will be supportive and positive about your finding a love connection. Until you are comfortable with the relationship yourselves, it might be best to date off the premises and be selective in telling friends. You can use humor in dealing with questions or comments from neighbors rather than answering direct queries: "Are you the dating police?"

The most difficult part of dating a neighbor comes when the relationship ends. Hopefully, as mature adults, you can remain friends, or at least be civil when you see each other. If you still have feelings for him, it will be difficult for you to see your former love with someone new. This seems the more critical issue, rather than the loss of privacy. Only you can answer whether you want to take some risk in finding love again.

*I think of myself as a considerate and friendly neighbor, and I am very distressed about how others on my floor who share my compactor room are not following the simplest rules about throwing away trash and recycling. I don't want to stir up hard feelings and say something to the culprits, but I am disgusted by the filth. What am I to do?*
—Grossed Out by Garbage,
Building 3

You have every reason to be concerned about the compactor room and any other infractions, such as leaving shopping carts in the hall overnight and at the elevator banks, or smoking in the stairwells. The health and safety of all residents is at stake. Yet confronting the possible culprits is a sensitive issue, even if you're sure who it is that doesn't throw their trash down the chute.

Several suggestions come to mind. Call the concierge desk and ask for a handyman to be sent up to remove large cartons or debris that's been left behind. If you know who is responsible, or if the mess is continual, the security office can be notified. Warning notes may be sent to offenders, and in extreme cases a lawyer's letter may be warranted. At times the family of a deceased neighbor may be cleaning out an apartment and may not know or care about the problems created by their debris. They could be charged for staff time or damage to the property.

The House and Grounds Committee is working on greater publicity about recycling and being a good neighbor—which also includes having your TVs and music playing at a respectful volume!

*I am perplexed by the behavior of my late husband's brother and his wife. When my*

*husband was alive, we socialized occasion-*
*ally since we live near one another. Since his*
*death last year, I never see them, nor do they*
*call me. When we run into each other they*
*say hello but never extend an invitation to*
*dinner, etc. I wonder if I have offended them*
*in some way and whether I should confront*
*them about this.*

—Abandoned In-Law,

Building 2

Confrontation is never a good policy since it implies an aggressive tactic. I would suggest that if this relationship is important to you, call your brother-in-law and sister-in-law and invite them over for lunch. You can tactfully tell them that you miss seeing them and that you wonder why you don't hear from them. Sometimes we misjudge a friendship that is based more on family duty or obligation than on genuine interest.

Sometimes a single woman poses a threat to a married couple who only socialize with other married couples. Also seeing you might reactivate your husband's brother's grief or his fears about his own future illness and death.

Since relationships are so complex, you will have to accept this change with your new widow status and move on if they don't include you in their life. You can feel comfortable that you have tried to reach out to them, and it is now up to them to determine if there is a basis to continue this relationship.

———

*I have been playing bridge with a neighbor for four years, and I now find that her memory is failing and her bridge skills are poor. I no longer want to play with her. How do I deal with this situation without hurting her feelings?*
—Ready to Burn the Bridge,
Building 3

This situation is complex, and one many of us may deal with, be it with a bridge, canasta, mah-jongg, golf, or tennis partner. Several issues and solutions come to mind. All must be handled sensitively and diplomatically. If your friend is unaware of his or her diminishing capacity, it will be more difficult to address. You can be honest and direct, and suggest the duplicate bridge game is becoming stressful for you and instead offer to play kitchen bridge with her. If this friendship is not important to you, you can make some excuse, and the relationship will probably end. If you want to continue the friendship, you might also be direct and say, "Let's have lunch or see a movie together," but tell her you have a new bridge partner who you met at a bridge course. While the friend may be hurt, you are also indicating your interest in continuing the friendship.

It might be more complicated if this bridge partner is a friend with whom you also socialize. You might be more willing to be tolerant and to continue to play with him or her because much more is at stake and you are not willing to risk ending the friendship. Of course there is the added concern about this person's diminishing capacity. As a good friend you might point this out to him or her so he or she can seek medical attention. A minor stroke or some other disorder might be the cause. In this way you can be a catalyst for directing your bridge partner to seek treatment.

It is necessary to take a risk so the situation improves and you do not feel like a victim. If you are suffering in silence, it may affect your health, or you may act out in some way—by being late or irritable with this partner.

⎯⎯⎯

*A neighbor recently lost her significant other—a man she lived with for ten years. Because I am also widowed she calls me daily and often cries. While I want to help her, this*

*situation is making me depressed. I don't want to turn her away, but I also don't want to be her therapist. What do I do?*
>                        —One Soaked Shoulder,
>                                Building 1

Because you too have grieved and can relate to her situation, it is difficult to turn her away. You can take several different approaches to this situation. Of course the first is the least helpful and honest: don't take her calls, or get off the phone as soon as possible, and she will get the message that you are not available to listen to her.

Secondly you can hear her out for a short time and then be honest and tell her this is not helping her or you. Direct her to a bereavement group, or to a therapist you or someone you know has consulted. Sometimes a person doesn't feel entitled to attending a bereavement group because they were not married to the deceased. This should not matter in a professionally run bereavement group, and you should encourage her to get the support she needs. If you can provide the name and telephone number of a group, that would be best.

Third encourage her to get involved in activities she enjoys, and offer to go out with her to a show or a museum. By distracting her you will not negate her feelings; you will offer your friendship and show her that even a grieving person can find pleasure in new pastimes. When she starts getting teary and morose, you can change the topic and thus not reinforce a depressive line of discussion.

# Health

This article is dedicated to my many friends, my family, and especially my love Chick Rudy, all of who have walked this journey with me and provided needed love and support.

A recent article in *The New York Times* (June 17, 2008) entitled "Cancer as a Disease, Not a Death Sentence" was of particular interest to me, since four years have passed since my cancer diagnosis.

With the initial diagnosis at stage 3C, I was able to ascertain the seriousness of my disease while never directly asking my doctor for a prognosis. In fact doctors have little way of determining who among their patients will survive and for how long!

While my cancer may never be cured, I have had a succession of treatments that have controlled the disease while providing me with a generally good quality of life. As described in the *Times* article, I have had a series of therapeutic approaches that work for a period of time, to be followed by another treatment that will stop the disease from progressing for a while. I have learned to live with a *stable* disease, which at times is referred to as a *chronic disease.*

My life has taken on a new normal that entails regular chemotherapy and frequent blood tests, body scans, and examinations. A level of anxiety continues to exist, especially before these diagnostic tests.

I'd never heard the term *sequential approach,* which was mentioned in the June 17 article, but I am living it. One specialist was quoted as saying the "ultimate goal was not to make this a chronic disease, but to keep patients alive long enough until we can find the right treatment for the right patient and cure the disease." Another doctor called the therapy "the hitch-hiker model," in which time is bought by going from point A to point B to point C and so on. This approach can continue indefinitely as long as new therapies become available and patients remain well enough to withstand the rigors of treatment.

My journey has included some rough times as far as hospitalizations and treatment side effects, but I am thankful for the wonderful care of the NYU Clinical Cancer Center staff, including Dr. John Curtin, Dr. David Fishman, and nurse practitioners Cathy Michalowski and Eileen Fusco. They have worked diligently and empathetically to get me to this point. As thankful as I am for the myriad treatments available, the side effects are debilitating. But my options are limited if I want to live.

The challenge of being a cancer survivor should not be devalued. Ovarian cancer is a chronic disease likened to diabetes, but that does not fully reflect the real picture. The word *chronic* connotes a disease that is easily managed, but that is not the case with ovarian cancer. Each recurrence brings many decisions, and remissions generally become shorter and shorter and bring with them concomitant side effects.

The journey is an arduous one, filled with many obstacles. Having family and friends to support me along the way is essential. My only hope is that continuing research will find the means to combat this deadly disease. That is the mission of the Varadi Ovarian Initiative for Cancer Education (VOICE), and we need your help to meet this goal.

*I've been living at North Shore Towers for two years and have met many people through the activities I enjoy. Most of these people are just acquaintances and not good friends. When I hear about someone's illness or a death in the family, I do not know if I should respond in*

*the way I usually do with old friends. I want
to be appropriate, yet be thoughtful. What do
you suggest?*

—Tactful Tina,

Building 1

Your question is a sensitive one that indicates you are a caring person who is somewhat insecure about the social graces in this large building complex. Apartment living often implies an impersonal relationship with neighbors who value their privacy. Yet North Shore Towers is unique—residents bond very quickly, and friendships flourish.

At least you might send a get well or condolence card and offer you help along with your telephone number, leaving it up to the acquaintance to respond to you. In this way you are not overstepping any boundaries. If you know a close friend of this acquaintance, you might ask if you could send over some soup or a special dish. Most people are most appreciative of this sort of gesture. Acts of loving kindness are the best gifts because through them you give of yourself.

At North Shore Towers, where there are many single people and some who don't drive, a lift to the doctor or help with chores is a most appreciated gift. If you are ever in need, you can be on the end of someone else's generosity. Giving in this way to someone in need—a mitzvah—is a reward in itself and makes you feel better. Don't worry too much about the appropriateness of your actions; just follow your good instincts.

———

*As a spouse of someone whose health is failing and who has a chronic condition, I find myself feeling guilty when I take time for myself and have someone else take responsibility for his care. Any suggestions?*
— Night and Day Nurse,
Building 3

The illness of a loved one—a spouse, parent, or child—creates tremendous stress, particularly if you are raised to be a nurturing caregiver. It is essential that you develop a strategy for how to meet the present challenges as well as how to plan ahead for various contingencies.

You have made an important step in acknowledging the complex feelings surrounding this issue. In addition to sadness about the deteriorating health of your spouse, there is resentment, anger, guilt, and feelings of helplessness. You also seem concerned and worried about the reactions of family and friends when you share care-taking responsibility with others.

Many have taken out insurance policies that pay for home health care, and if that is your situation, take advantage of it and hire someone to assist you. Even if you must pay out of pocket at this time, it is important to have someone to share this responsibility with you. While family members might be able to help, it is unrealistic to expect those with responsibilities of their own to provide the consistency you will need. Eldercare lawyers and social workers can give you direction for planning ahead. Perhaps consider assisted living or a nursing home facility.

It is important to explore all community resources that can provide respite care. We are fortunate to live close to facilities like Parker Geriatric Center and the Samuel Field Y, which have day programs. These centers also have support groups for caregivers and can provide individual counseling help.

While participating in groups may not be comfortable for you initially, they may help you to establish a support network through which you can meet new friends for social activities. Right now you are no longer part of a couple for social activities, and you are not a widow either. Old friends can offer support, but they are not experiencing the ambiguity of your situation and may not be able to empathize fully with you.

It is essential that you try to diminish the effects of stress by enjoying activities that bring you pleasure. Here at the NST, there is the health club, the pool, cards, meetings, book clubs, etc. Local colleges and religious institutions have courses that can provide educational and spiritual comfort. Outings with friends and vacations can take you away physically from the day-to-day caregiving responsibilities, and you do need to give yourself permission to take care of yourself without guilt. Your health can suffer under the stress of your present living situation, and you need to do everything necessary to feel good physically, emotionally, and spiritually. The caregiver must take of herself too.

How does an incurable disease change your life?

I've been introspective this last week after attending funerals for two women in my ovarian cancer support group. In some ways I've been luckier than some ovarian cancer survivors; I've gone through five years of treatment and still have had a good quality of life. I am able to exercise, play cards, go to the theater and museums, have dinners out with friends, etc. I do restrict my travel to stays in Florida and local weekend getaways, and I miss the experience of national and international travel. But the thought of being away from my doctors and hospitals makes me fearful, and I am not willing to sacrifice my comfort level for new adventures.

I have simplified my life in some ways, such as

not making social plans in advance most of the time. Since I am unable to predict how I might feel on any particular day, it is easier this way and causes less tension for me. I don't have to worry about disappointing friends and changing plans at the last minute.

Psychologically a cloud hangs over my head, and many emotional ups and downs have prevented me from having the carefree existence I wish for. I have learned to be more patient and less anxious about certain aspects of treatment.

Most important has been a change in my general attitude—namely I now don't sweat the small stuff. This means putting daily events in perspective and focusing on the big picture. A broken nail, a dent in the car, and even a downturn in the stock market no longer seem so important.

I place more value on the love and support of family and friends and am thankful for calls to inquire about my health and for small gestures of caring.

In fact I am grateful for every day that I feel fine!

As a psychologist I have always been interested in helping others, but now I give of myself in a different way—by being open about my struggles. I no longer need to be seen as invulnerable.

While being nonjudgmental is part of my professional training, I am now even more accepting. As the teenagers say, "Whatever." That too has become my mantra. I have become more open to numerous ideas and to people who share different philosophies. I can disagree without being disagreeable, and I try to find positive qualities in all people.

My involvement with VOICE, a foundation that funds research into early detection of ovarian cancer, has been one way of making lemonade out of lemons. I have become a vocal advocate in this area and am not fearful of expressing my views on various matters. I have finally learned to assert myself.

Difficult times, while stressful, can make you stronger and can lead to positive changes in attitude and ways of living. It feels good to reach out to others. Paying it forward, as Oprah says, can be the most gratifying to those who give. You receive from giving to others!

*What is my obligation to my neighbor, who I don't know by name, if she appears ill? I was in the arcade in front of a shop when I noticed a lady was slumped over sitting on her walker and apparently alone.*

—Good Samaritan,
Building 2

This situation is not uncommon here at the North Shore Towers and deserves attention. Minimally it seems you should notify security about this woman so emergency services can be provided. Security's telephone number is (718) 423-7990, and it should be posted at each vendor's telephone in case you don't remember it. Stay with the woman until someone from security arrives on the scene, but it's not incumbent on you to remain until paramedics arrive.

If you or someone else knows the building the woman lives in and her name, you might also consider contacting that building's concierge or the management office in case they have an emergency contact number for a family member who should be notified.

The importance of having emergency information on file can't be stressed enough. Unfortunately it is often left to our wonderful NST staff to contact family members even in non-emergency situations.

*What is my obligation to a friend or acquaintance when I recognize her health is failing?*
—A Friend to Friends in Need,
Building 1

This is a far more complicated question than the previous one, yet addressing it might help to prevent an emergency situation like the prior one.

The role you take in such a situation depends on your closeness to this friend and your willingness to take some risk in the relationship. If you discuss health issues and doctor's visits, you could encourage your friend to see her doctor and point out—diplomatically—anything health-wise you have noticed recently. That might include her dozing during canasta or forgetting what she ordered for dinner.

If this friend has symptoms such as confusion, this can create difficulty in the discussion. If you know her children, you should consider speaking with them about the situation. Often children are unaware of such problems or in denial. Accepting the declining health of a parent must inevitably lead to planning for needed services like a health aide or an assisted living facility.

In the event that you don't contact a family member and your friend is aware of her declining health and her needs, you might suggest she hire someone to assist her. Many qualified health aides work at NST and can assist your friend in finding someone. Unfortunately, at times, an aide who works for someone else feels it's her responsibility to assist when in the presence of this person, and that is an improper situation—especially if the aide is your aide.

Our caring and concern for our neighbors and friends is what makes us human and what makes NST such a unique family community.

———

Many thanks to those of you who have called or spoken to me about August's column. If it has inspired you or touched you in some way, that was one of my goals. It was also helpful to me to write it.

During these years of illness, I have learned many lessons. One is that you must be your own advocate with regard to the medical system. Many of us have grown up with great respect and awe for doctors, which generally meant not questioning what we were told. We followed doctors' orders regarding diagnostic tests and various treatments.

There has been a significant shift in the behavior of patients now; some of this is due to various rights movements, some due to the abundance of information on the Internet and media and the openness of friends about medical issues. We are generally better informed, and most doctors have shifted in their interactions with their patients. Now we don't accept their paternalistic attitudes, and as consumers we are apt to change doctors until we find someone who is willing to accept us as partners in determining our care.

For me the more information I have, the more

comfortable I am. I like to read scan reports (even if I don't understand them). I have copies of all my blood work results, and I keep a detailed diary of my treatments. I ask many questions, and I let the medical people know about my concerns and preferences.

I realize this is not everyone's style. There are those who feel more comfortable not knowing and those who don't even seek the opinion of a doctor when they are experiencing symptoms. While sometimes symptoms disappear after a while, being an ostrich with your head in the sand often is dangerous!

In my case only two weeks passed between the evening I could not button my slacks and my abdominal surgery. If my gynecologist had not been on vacation, that time would have been shorter.

I urge everyone to take the initiative when your health is concerned and even seek second and third opinions if you are displeased with your primary doctor's response. Your life should be in your hands!

As an aside, I'm sometimes asked, and am sometimes confused myself, about HIPAA privacy practices. We are all given HIPAA forms at all doctors' and dentists' offices and are even asked to sign forms that acknowledge we have received the notices.

My understanding is that this is a way of protecting patient confidentiality—i.e., so that information about you can only be given to others with your permission. Obviously you agree that insurance companies can receive information, as can other agencies deemed necessary for your protection.

Medical establishments interpret this in various ways. Most doctors' offices call out your name; some have you sign in when you arrive. But the content of your medical condition is confidential. Signs in hospital elevators caution doctors about discussing medical matters in public settings, and pharmacies request that you stand back when someone is at the counter—all to protect your privacy.

Informal issues of confidentiality also come to mind, whether they're medical or nonmedical. As a psychologist I know the ethics regarding the patients I treat. However, for all of us, there is no clear line when someone shares personal information. Some people are more open while others are private. It is best to ask if shared information should remain confidential.

I interpret HIPAA in another way—namely that your health information must be disclosed to you! I plan on researching this further. I like to have lab results and other test findings in hand, so I can read them before my doctor calls to discuss them. Call me a control freak, but it's my body we're talking about.

*I have many friends with developing health problems. I offer advice, which my friends generally ignore. This is very frustrating. Any suggestions?*
—Two Cents and Then Some,
Building 3

Your friends are fortunate to have you as a caring, good listener when they are anxious about their health. It sounds as if they may not be asking for advice, however. Sometimes friends just need an opportunity to vent their feelings about their worries and medical concerns.

Most people, like you, feel at a loss as to what to say or do when hearing about health issues. They generally make suggestions about tests, medicines, or doctors. Sometimes they give the names of others to talk to who have similar health problems.

Some of these friends may even refuse to see doctors or take their medications regularly, which makes it more difficult for you to have an effective conversation.

In these scenarios you have limited choices. On the one hand, you can continue to listen and be frustrated when your suggestions are ignored. On the other hand, you can take a direct, tough-love approach by telling your friends you are not willing to listen to their complaints unless they take appropriate medical actions.

The latter approach is the better course because you will be less frustrated, and hopefully your friends will get the help they need.

———

*A dear friend became seriously ill several months ago, and I feel uncomfortable calling her since I don't know what to say. Any suggestions?*
—At a Loss for Words,
Building 3

Your discomfort in the face of your friend's illness is not uncommon. On one level it is distressing to focus on the illness of a contemporary because it arouses in you feelings about your own vulnerability. As we age we often become more worried about our mortality.

On another level you are powerless to affect any change concerning your friend's health. This creates a feeling of helplessness in you because we are used to offering help in the form of solutions.

However help can be offered in other ways. The best approach is to call and ask your friend how you can be of assistance. Depending upon her openness, she may make suggestions like assisting with shopping (food, books, etc.), preparing her favorite soup, helping with calls or paperwork, or accompanying her to a doctor appointment.

Often people with illness don't want to talk about their treatments or prognoses, so you need not be worried about difficult issues. If your friend feels like discussing her medical condition, you can listen and say something supportive, such as, "I know you're going through a difficult time." While we often want to be reassuring and say, "You'll be fine," it is best not to offer what may be false hope.

If your friend gets very specific about her illness, and it makes you feel uncomfortable, you can try to change the topic or be more direct and say such information is hard for you to hear.

Your friend will appreciate your reaching out to her on your terms. It's preferable to cutting off communication, as you have!

———

*Please help! I live fifteen minutes from my folks, and my sister lives forty-five minutes away in New Jersey. We are both retirees and married. It has been my responsibility to look in on my parents regularly, but they are now ill, and I find my days busy with taking them to doctor appointments. In addition my*

*sister continues to advise me on what to do. I
feel she is not sharing this burden, and I am
resentful. Any suggestions?*
 —The Good—and Busy—Daughter,
 Building 2

You are in a difficult situation that many of us face. The least you would want from your sister is a little appreciation for the efforts involved in the care of your parents. If she lived farther away and was working, you might be more understanding of her difficulty in sharing responsibilities.

You are also thinking ahead to when these demands on you will increase, and you must plan ahead and include your sister in this important discussion. Your spouse's feelings must also be considered, and he too may have responsibilities to aging parents.

The discussion with your sister may include having her commit to specific days to visit and be involved with doctors, etc., or having your parents spend time at her home. She may also consider paying for an aide who can drive your parents to doctors and assist them, so you can be relieved of some responsibility. Longer-range planning may include moving your parents to a facility where services are provided for them. The financial aspect of this must also be part of the discussion.

In every family there seems to be one sibling who takes on the caregiver role more than others; sometimes it's the women rather than the men. Resentments that build impact all other aspects of sibling relationships. It is far better to clear the air with a proactive discussion so the relationship doesn't become toxic.

# Money Makes
# the World Go 'Round

*At our Thanksgiving dinner, my sister-in-law mentioned she and her husband couldn't afford to buy their dream retirement home in Florida. She hinted that her parents should buy it for them now, since my husband, who is her brother, has plenty of money. She has always been jealous of our lifestyle, but I think she's way off base. My husband said nothing in response. Shall I say something to my husband or his parents about this?*
—What's Mine Is Mine,
Building 3

Say something only if you want World War III. Realistically, as a sister-in-law you have no standing in this matter, and it would be best to stay away from a discussion with your husband or in-laws. When it comes to money matters, even the closest of families can go to war.

Your sister-in-law's jealousy is not easy to deal with,

and if in fact you are more affluent, it would be best to be discreet about your vacation plans, expenditures, etc. Some families help out financially or give generous gifts, if they can afford to regularly, as a way of dealing with estate taxes. Your sister-in-law's suggesting she get part of her inheritance early isn't so uncommon.

Issues relating to inheritances of money, property, jewelry, etc. are often the arena in which sibling rivalries emerge. Sometimes parents discuss this with their adult children when they write their wills, and at other times only upon their deaths do their children face these situations. Sometimes the siblings share inheritances equally, and in other families it may be based upon need.

It is your husband's responsibility to discuss this with his parents and sister if it is of concern to him. It would be foolish of you to interject your opinion since there is no winning in this scenario. Your husband may not be concerned about equity and may be more generous of heart than you are. Some soul-searching by you might reveal your own feelings and attitudes toward your siblings.

———

*You have discussed money issues in this column before, but as a woman in a long-term second marriage this issue rears its*

*head over and over again. For example when one of my children needs a loan, I must discuss it with my spouse, who often feels it is not fair to give one child more than another, whether natural or stepchild. What is fair? I don't like having to ask for permission to do what I think is needed in a situation. Any suggestions?*
—Loan Officer at Mom's Bank,
Building 3

Having to ask for permission from your spouse is obviously what is most troubling in the relationship. It also has implications as to how money matters in general are handled. If you have your own funds, this is less irksome. Your sense of independence will depend on whether you have earned income during the marriage. Independence in money matters makes it possible for you to follow your heart, perhaps without even discussing it with your husband.

Fairness about money is irrelevant in my opinion. Your children have different needs based upon their incomes, family sizes, and values. A small monetary gift to one child may mean a prized vacation while the same amount may mean a trinket for the sports car of another child.

Families with stepchildren are most complicated. Remember money means more than cash; it may involve competition and feelings of being loved. Until everyone reaches a level of total unselfishness toward and acceptance of the stepparents and stepchildren, you can expect these issues to come to the fore.

In the best of all worlds, you and your spouse will work this problem out—perhaps with the aid of accountants and lawyers, since upon the death of one spouse, dividing assets will become a major headache. Money should not be the major focus of relationships.

―――

*In-law relationships are a great challenge in general, but more so when a family business is involved. My son-in-law and brother-in-law work in my husband's business, and now there's talk of bringing my nephew in as well. Any suggestions?*

—All in the Family,
Building 3

Your concern is well founded, but I am unclear whether your husband, who has the most at stake, is as worried as you are. Often men are more matter-of-fact in these situations, and we women obsess over such interpersonal matters.

Your husband's prior and present family experiences

and his personality play larges part in how another family member can be incorporated into the business. For example your husband may have worked with his father and brothers, and all went smoothly, with each having a clear role and responsibilities. It is unclear if your brother-in-law is your husband's brother or the husband of your sister. Also, did your husband feel obligated to have your brother-in-law work for him, or is the brother-in-law a vital asset to the business? Likewise how does your son-in-law feel about having your nephew join the business? Jealousy can easily surface in such situations.

It may be a generalization, but in-law relationships between women appear more contentious. In the TV series *Everybody Loves Raymond*, the mother-in-law and daughter-in-law relationship is characterized by extreme competitiveness and a difficulty sharing Raymond. The humor in the situation, while exaggerated, highlights a relationship that often is not easy.

When business and financial matters are added to the mix, you may be correct in foreseeing difficulties. One is often cautioned about doing any business with family or friends, because a lot is at stake if things go badly.

One suggestion would be to think through all concerns in advance, and perhaps consult with an attorney or accountant. The specific job description, with salary, should be written down. Also consider a trial period to see if this is the right business decision for all concerned.

Overall, I believe, careful planning and discussion beforehand can help to eliminate potential problems. With family we often must work harder at resolving differences, and combining family and business presents a great challenge.

———

*I have been married for more than forty years and have always been in charge of our money. I've paid all the bills, including restaurant tabs. As a traditional stay-at-home mom who didn't work outside the home, I still have to defend myself to friends who ask how much allowance I give my husband. Any suggestions?*
                          —A Nose for Numbers,
                                  Building 3

I commend you on finding a solution for money matters that obviously works for both you and your husband. As you may know, conflicts over money can be one of the most serious battlefields in a marriage, often leading to divorce. Since each spouse comes from a family with different role models and values about how money is treated, it is wonderful that you and your husband have little conflict in this area.

Money represents many different things: power, control, security, and independence, to name a few. In a marriage there needs to be a balance of power as well as sensitivity to each other's needs. Compromise and negotiation take place when dealing with both the important and the mundane in a marriage. Money matters are often very complex. Do we have separate as well as joint accounts and credit cards? Who pays for what? Can you spend on luxuries and extras without consulting your partner? How do you manage if values about money are very different?

Early on in your marriage, you and your husband found a model that works for you and is not threatened by your controlling the purse strings. You seem comfortable as a liberated woman in this arena. Showing some humor to friends who tease you would work the best. Say, "He's afraid of leaving all his money to OTB."

*I am divorced and the father of two twenty-plus sons. The youngest is graduating from college and just informed me that he plans on going to law school in the fall. His older*

*brother is now thinking of dental school. Both
boys went to expensive private colleges, and
I paid. I had not counted on this additional
financial burden but am being made to feel
guilty if I don't help. Any advice?*

—Paid My Dues,

Building 1

The matter of money again. In this situation money seems to represent love, caring, and commitment. In some sense your sons may be testing your love for them through their unilateral decisions about graduate school. It sounds like the graduating son applied and was accepted to law school without discussing this plan with you, leading me to believe your relationship is somewhat estranged.

How did he expect to pay for it? Scholarships, loans, and money from his mother or other family? This seems like an opportune time to have a discussion about what you want to offer your son without feeling guilt or anger. You can show your love and concern by helping to negotiate a plan that is realistic, such as a deferred loan that he will repay after graduation. You might confer with your accountant about educational tax deductions, but don't feel blackmailed in this matter. If you do you will feel more resentful, and your relationship will suffer as a result.

What is most interesting is your older son's recent decision about dental school. His decision has the flavor of sibling rivalry and the "me too" syndrome. It appears he is testing you to see if he will get the same as his brother. Since his plans seem less specific, a talk with him about what he needs from you in more general terms seems warranted.

While your sons have confronted you with a surprising financial dilemma, take this opportunity to develop a more adult relationship with them. Their reactions to your divorce still need to be worked on. They seem to be struggling with decisions about themselves and their futures and need your support at this time.

*I have been living at North Shore Towers with my significant other for ten years, and he owns the apartment. While I get along well with his children, I fear I will be dispossessed if something happens to him, for example if he goes to a nursing home. What do you suggest?*

—Seeking Security,
Building 1

Many residents may share your concern, since many couples choose to live together rather than marry in their later years. This usually involves the children and the state, and the co-op is now a significant part of the estate. My advice is to consult a lawyer with your partner if he is amenable to it. I expect some provisions can be made in his will to protect you upon his death, but an intermediary plan like a nursing home might not be addressed thoughtfully by anyone. This requires legal advice.

Some couples have had their co-op retitled in the name of both partners, and they've worked out financial aspects with the knowledge of their children. Again legal intervention is needed in this scenario. You are wise to consider this when you are both healthy and under the pressure of some imminent decision. While you have a good relationship with your partner's children, they have finances to be concerned about and might not be as beneficent as you would like. It is necessary to take whatever steps are necessary to protect yourself in this situation.

———

*My younger brother, who is married with children, always has financial problems, and I've helped him out in the past. Now my*

*husband tells me I am a pushover and seems
to object to my inclination to keep helping my
brother. Any suggestions?*
                              —Dependable Donna,
                                    Building 3

It is admirable that you care for and are able financially to help your brother and his family. Your acts of
generosity should give you pleasure and not cause you
to feel guilty or cause conflict between you and your
husband.

While you haven't said specifically how you help,
I suggest outright gifts rather than loans that may
never be repaid. Don't expect to change your brother's
spending habits, and don't have strings attached to
giving. This will only create conflict and bad feelings.
You might also consider establishing a college fund for
his children, which provides a tax advantage for you
and an important asset for them.

With regard to your husband's concern, it is
important that he understands you don't feel exploited
by your brother—rather you feel proud and happy that
you can help. Since you are a giving person, your husband should feel confident that you will be there for
him and other family members when there is a need
emotionally, physically, or financially.

In most marriages, after expenses are taken care of,

there is discretionary money that each spouse may use as he or she determines fit. If you choose to send money to your brother rather than buy the latest handbag, then that should be your decision. While I don't encourage lying or deceiving your husband, there is no reason to discuss the details of your philanthropy, especially when your brother does something that disappoints.

———

*I am concerned about disclosing information about my financial assets to my children, but my advisors suggest I meet with them now to plan in the event of my disability or death. What do you think?*
                              —Taking It to the Grave,
                                        Building 1

An underlying aspect of this question deals with your discomfort about the future. To confront our own mortality is surely difficult, but it's something that needs to be done.

Your children need to be involved in several ways that concern health and financial matters. Your advisors—your lawyer, accountant, and/or financial planner—have experience with these issues and are correct in prompting you to begin an open dialogue. It is never too early to start such a discussion.

Your children may be just as uncomfortable as you are about having this type of talk, so you might consider having one of your advisors participate in or run the meeting. An outsider can serve as both a moderator and a source of technical information.

The children should know where important documents are kept, and they should know your wishes as stated in your living will. They should know if they are named as your health care proxies, and they should have copies of the document. Your concerns about declining health should also be addressed, and together you can explore options for your care.

There may be sensitive issues to be discussed, and you and your children may not be in agreement. However having such a meeting can open an ongoing dialogue that hopefully will resolve all issues eventually.

Many people share stories of families that are torn apart after the death of a parent. Sometimes these matters can be resolved with earlier compromises that help to prevent such problems later on.

I suggest you bite the bullet and think about the future. While it might be difficult at first, planning ahead is a legacy you want to leave your family.

# About the Author

Marilyn Meyrow Varadi was born in the Midwood section of Brooklyn to parents who placed a strong emphasis on education, inspiring her and her brother to earn advanced degrees. She attended Midwood High and Harpur College, State University of Binghamton. She received a BA from Brooklyn College and a master's degree in school psychology from City College. After a clinical internship at the Staten Island Mental Health Center, she began pursuing a doctorate at NYU and received a PhD from NYU. She also earned a New York State certification in educational administration.

Marilyn became a licensed psychologist and certified school psychologist. She had a thirty-year career with the New York City Board of Education and established a private practice specializing in family issues and relationships, with a subspecialty in infertility counseling.

Marilyn rose to become supervisor of school psychologists with the NYC Board of Education. Upon her retirement she became an associate professor, joining the adjunct faculty of the school psychology departments of both New York University and Queens College.

In 1968 she married John Varadi, a Hungarian refugee; they have a daughter, Lisa. They lived in Manhattan before moving to Great Neck and Westhampton, Long Island. After John's death in 1991, Marilyn met Chick Rudy, and they were together for almost twenty years.

For many years Marilyn was not only an educator and a psychologist but an advocate for children and parents. She has served on the board of Resolve, a national infertility organization, and ran support groups for infertile couples. She appeared on radio and in the press regarding to her involvement with and education of couples about the emotional consequences of infertility.

In her spare time, Marilyn enjoyed bridge, golf, and semi-retirement. The foundation established the Marilyn Varadi Research Fellowship for Ovarian Cancer Research at the NYU Medical Center in 2007.

Marilyn lost her battle with ovarian cancer on September 1, 2010, after a six-year fight that included 160 chemotherapy treatments. "I would define my credo as being generally optimistic: an outlook that focuses on positive thinking," she wrote in her final column for the *Tower Times* that summer. "What has helped to take the focus off myself and allowed me not to be mired in self-pity has been my ability to reach out to others in similar situations. That we are not alone in our lostness may be the essence of caring."

In remembrance of Dr. Varadi, her family suggests contributing to the Varadi Ovarian Initiative for Cancer Education (VOICE), Mount Sinai School of Medicine, 1176 Fifth Avenue KP-9, New York, NY 10029.